Anxiety Journal

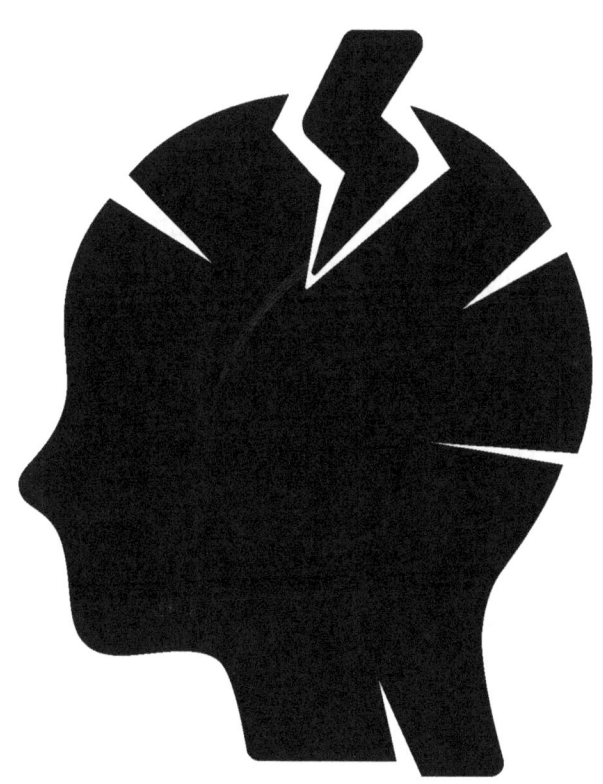

© Copyright 2021 - All rights reserved.

You may not reproduce, duplicate or send the contents of this book without direct written permission from the author. You cannot hereby despite any circumstance blame the publisher or hold him or her to legal responsibility for any reparation, compensations, or monetary forfeiture owing to the information included herein, either in a direct or an indirect way.

Legal Notice: This book has copyright protection. You can use the book for personal purpose. You should not sell, use, alter, distribute, quote, take excerpts or paraphrase in part or whole the material contained in this book without obtaining the permission of the author first.

Disclaimer Notice: You must take note that the information in this document is for casual reading and entertainment purposes only.
We have made every attempt to provide accurate, up to date and reliable information. We do not express or imply guarantees of any kind. The persons who read admit that the writer is not occupied in giving legal, financial, medical or other advice. We put this book content by sourcing various places.

Please consult a licensed professional before you try any techniques shown in this book. By going through this document, the book lover comes to an agreement that under no situation is the author accountable for any forfeiture, direct or indirect, which they may incur because of the use of material contained in this document, including, but not limited to, — errors, omissions, or inaccuracies.

THIS ANXIETY JOURNAL BELONGS TO

_____

_____

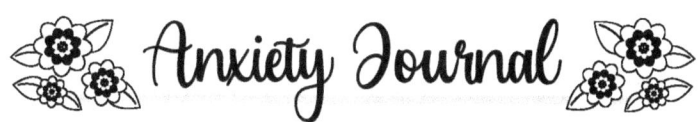

DATE   TIME

PLACE   SOURCE OF ANXIETY

PHYSICAL SENSATIONS

NEGATIVE BELIEVES

ABOUT SITUATION ....
....

ABOUT YOUSELF ....
....

WHAT FACTS DO YOU KNOW ARE TRUE?

ABOUT SITUATION ....
....

ABOUT YOUSELF ....
....

WHAT HAPPENED?

....
....

HOW DID IT MAKE YOU FEEL?

....
....

HOW DID YOU REACT?

....
....

WHAT HELPS YOU SOOTHE YOUR ANXIETY?

....
....

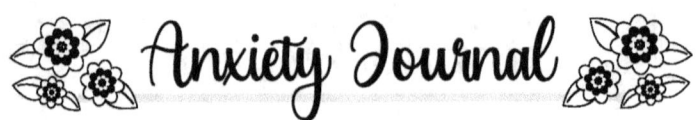

Anxiety Journal

DATE .... **TIME** ....

PLACE .... **SOURCE OF ANXIETY** ....

PHYSICAL SENSATIONS ....

NEGATIVE BELIEVES

ABOUT SITUATION ....
....

ABOUT YOUSELF ....
....

WHAT FACTS DO YOU KNOW ARE TRUE?

ABOUT SITUATION ....
....

ABOUT YOUSELF ....
....

WHAT HAPPENED?

....
....

HOW DID IT MAKE YOU FEEL?

....
....

HOW DID YOU REACT?

....
....

WHAT HELPS YOU SOOTHE YOUR ANXIETY?

....
....

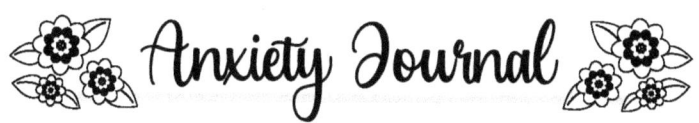

Anxiety Journal

DATE .... TIME ....

PLACE .... SOURCE OF ANXIETY ....

PHYSICAL SENSATIONS ....

NEGATIVE BELIEVES

ABOUT SITUATION ....
....

ABOUT YOUSELF ....
....

WHAT FACTS DO YOU KNOW ARE TRUE?

ABOUT SITUATION ....
....

ABOUT YOUSELF ....
....

WHAT HAPPENED?

....
....

HOW DID IT MAKE YOU FEEL?

....
....

HOW DID YOU REACT?

....
....

WHAT HELPS YOU SOOTHE YOUR ANXIETY?

....
....

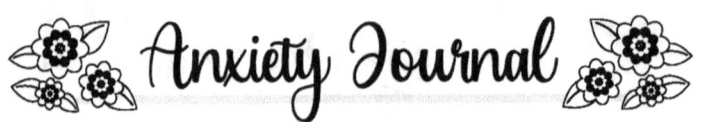

Anxiety Journal

DATE   **TIME**

PLACE   **SOURCE OF ANXIETY**

PHYSICAL SENSATIONS

NEGATIVE BELIEVES

ABOUT SITUATION ....
....

ABOUT YOUSELF ....
....

WHAT FACTS DO YOU KNOW ARE TRUE?

ABOUT SITUATION ....
....

ABOUT YOUSELF ....
....

WHAT HAPPENED?

....
....

HOW DID IT MAKE YOU FEEL?

....
....

HOW DID YOU REACT?

....
....

WHAT HELPS YOU SOOTHE YOUR ANXIETY?

....
....

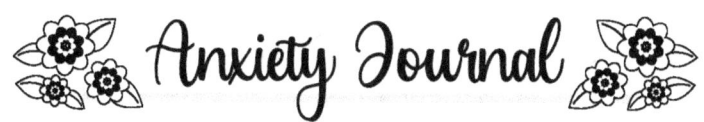

DATE TIME

PLACE SOURCE OF ANXIETY

PHYSICAL SENSATIONS

NEGATIVE BELIEVES

ABOUT SITUATION ....
....

ABOUT YOUSELF ....
....

WHAT FACTS DO YOU KNOW ARE TRUE?

ABOUT SITUATION ....
....

ABOUT YOUSELF ....
....

WHAT HAPPENED?

....
....

HOW DID IT MAKE YOU FEEL?

....
....

HOW DID YOU REACT?

....
....

WHAT HELPS YOU SOOTHE YOUR ANXIETY?

....
....

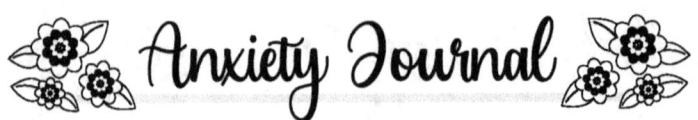

Anxiety Journal

DATE .... TIME ....

PLACE .... SOURCE OF ANXIETY ....

PHYSICAL SENSATIONS ....

NEGATIVE BELIEVES

ABOUT SITUATION ....
....

ABOUT YOUSELF ....
....

WHAT FACTS DO YOU KNOW ARE TRUE?

ABOUT SITUATION ....
....

ABOUT YOUSELF ....
....

WHAT HAPPENED?

....
....

HOW DID IT MAKE YOU FEEL?

....
....

HOW DID YOU REACT?

....
....

WHAT HELPS YOU SOOTHE YOUR ANXIETY?

....
....

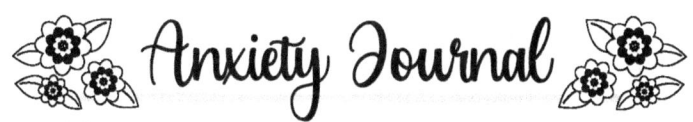

DATE   TIME

PLACE   SOURCE OF ANXIETY

PHYSICAL SENSATIONS

NEGATIVE BELIEVES

ABOUT SITUATION ....

ABOUT YOUSELF ....

WHAT FACTS DO YOU KNOW ARE TRUE?

ABOUT SITUATION ....

ABOUT YOUSELF ....

WHAT HAPPENED?

....

HOW DID IT MAKE YOU FEEL?

....

HOW DID YOU REACT?

....

WHAT HELPS YOU SOOTHE YOUR ANXIETY?

....

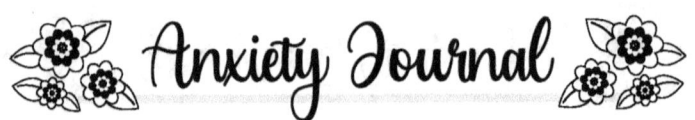
Anxiety Journal

DATE _____ TIME _____

PLACE _____ SOURCE OF ANXIETY _____

PHYSICAL SENSATIONS _____

NEGATIVE BELIEVES
ABOUT SITUATION ....
....
ABOUT YOUSELF ....
....

WHAT FACTS DO YOU KNOW ARE TRUE?
ABOUT SITUATION ....
....
ABOUT YOUSELF ....
....

WHAT HAPPENED?
....
....

HOW DID IT MAKE YOU FEEL?
....
....

HOW DID YOU REACT?
....
....

WHAT HELPS YOU SOOTHE YOUR ANXIETY?
....
....

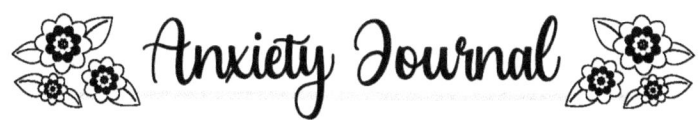

Anxiety Journal

DATE .... TIME ....

PLACE .... SOURCE OF ANXIETY ....

PHYSICAL SENSATIONS ....

NEGATIVE BELIEVES

ABOUT SITUATION ....
....

ABOUT YOUSELF ....
....

WHAT FACTS DO YOU KNOW ARE TRUE?

ABOUT SITUATION ....
....

ABOUT YOUSELF ....
....

WHAT HAPPENED?

....
....

HOW DID IT MAKE YOU FEEL?

....
....

HOW DID YOU REACT?

....
....

WHAT HELPS YOU SOOTHE YOUR ANXIETY?

....
....

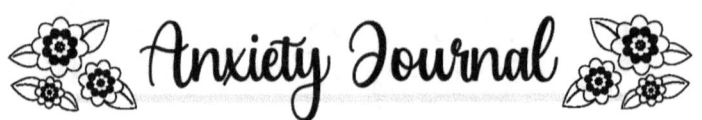

Anxiety Journal

DATE .... TIME ....

PLACE .... SOURCE OF ANXIETY ....

PHYSICAL SENSATIONS ....

NEGATIVE BELIEVES

ABOUT SITUATION ....
....

ABOUT YOUSELF ....
....

WHAT FACTS DO YOU KNOW ARE TRUE?

ABOUT SITUATION ....
....

ABOUT YOUSELF ....
....

WHAT HAPPENED?

....
....

HOW DID IT MAKE YOU FEEL?

....
....

HOW DID YOU REACT?

....
....

WHAT HELPS YOU SOOTHE YOUR ANXIETY?

....
....

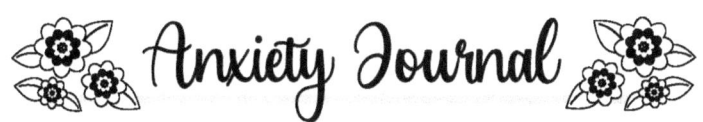

Anxiety Journal

DATE TIME

PLACE SOURCE OF ANXIETY

PHYSICAL SENSATIONS

NEGATIVE BELIEVES

ABOUT SITUATION ....
....

ABOUT YOUSELF ....
....

WHAT FACTS DO YOU KNOW ARE TRUE?

ABOUT SITUATION ....
....

ABOUT YOUSELF ....
....

WHAT HAPPENED?

....
....

HOW DID IT MAKE YOU FEEL?

....
....

HOW DID YOU REACT?

....
....

WHAT HELPS YOU SOOTHE YOUR ANXIETY?

....
....

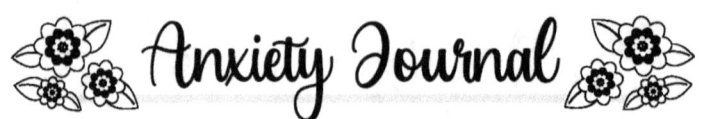

DATE .... TIME ....
PLACE .... SOURCE OF ANXIETY ....
PHYSICAL SENSATIONS ....

NEGATIVE BELIEVES

ABOUT SITUATION ....
....

ABOUT YOUSELF ....
....

WHAT FACTS DO YOU KNOW ARE TRUE?

ABOUT SITUATION ....
....

ABOUT YOUSELF ....
....

WHAT HAPPENED?

....
....

HOW DID IT MAKE YOU FEEL?

....
....

HOW DID YOU REACT?

....
....

WHAT HELPS YOU SOOTHE YOUR ANXIETY?

....
....

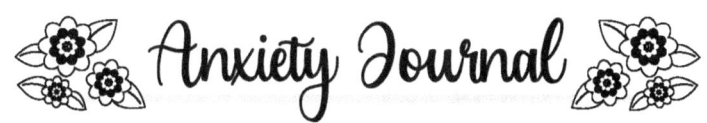

Anxiety Journal

DATE   **TIME**

PLACE   **SOURCE OF ANXIETY**

PHYSICAL SENSATIONS

NEGATIVE BELIEVES

ABOUT SITUATION ....
....

ABOUT YOUSELF ....
....

WHAT FACTS DO YOU KNOW ARE TRUE?

ABOUT SITUATION ....
....

ABOUT YOUSELF ....
....

WHAT HAPPENED?

....
....

HOW DID IT MAKE YOU FEEL?

....
....

HOW DID YOU REACT?

....
....

WHAT HELPS YOU SOOTHE YOUR ANXIETY?

....
....

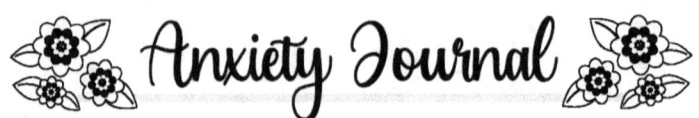

Anxiety Journal

DATE .... **TIME** ....

PLACE .... **SOURCE OF ANXIETY** ....

PHYSICAL SENSATIONS ....

NEGATIVE BELIEVES

ABOUT SITUATION ....
....

ABOUT YOUSELF ....
....

WHAT FACTS DO YOU KNOW ARE TRUE?

ABOUT SITUATION ....
....

ABOUT YOUSELF ....
....

WHAT HAPPENED?

....
....

HOW DID IT MAKE YOU FEEL?

....
....

HOW DID YOU REACT?

....
....

WHAT HELPS YOU SOOTHE YOUR ANXIETY?

....
....

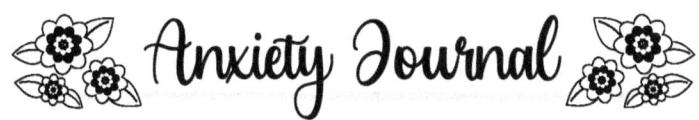

Anxiety Journal

DATE TIME

PLACE SOURCE OF ANXIETY

PHYSICAL SENSATIONS

NEGATIVE BELIEVES

ABOUT SITUATION ....

....

ABOUT YOUSELF ....

....

WHAT FACTS DO YOU KNOW ARE TRUE?

ABOUT SITUATION ....

....

ABOUT YOUSELF ....

....

WHAT HAPPENED?

....

....

HOW DID IT MAKE YOU FEEL?

....

....

HOW DID YOU REACT?

....

....

WHAT HELPS YOU SOOTHE YOUR ANXIETY?

....

....

Anxiety Journal

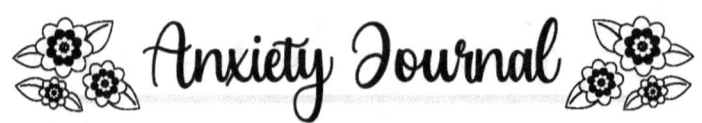

DATE .... **TIME** ....

PLACE .... **SOURCE OF ANXIETY** ....

PHYSICAL SENSATIONS ....

NEGATIVE BELIEVES

ABOUT SITUATION ....
....

ABOUT YOUSELF ....
....

WHAT FACTS DO YOU KNOW ARE TRUE?

ABOUT SITUATION ....
....

ABOUT YOUSELF ....
....

WHAT HAPPENED?

....
....

HOW DID IT MAKE YOU FEEL?

....
....

HOW DID YOU REACT?

....
....

WHAT HELPS YOU SOOTHE YOUR ANXIETY?

....
....

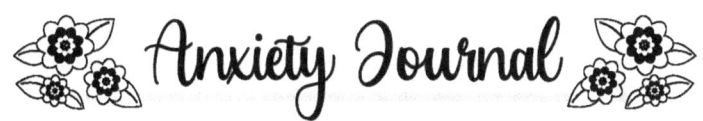

Anxiety Journal

DATE   TIME

PLACE   SOURCE OF ANXIETY

PHYSICAL SENSATIONS

NEGATIVE BELIEVES

ABOUT SITUATION ....

ABOUT YOUSELF ....

WHAT FACTS DO YOU KNOW ARE TRUE?

ABOUT SITUATION ....

ABOUT YOUSELF ....

WHAT HAPPENED?

....
....

HOW DID IT MAKE YOU FEEL?

....
....

HOW DID YOU REACT?

....
....

WHAT HELPS YOU SOOTHE YOUR ANXIETY?

....
....

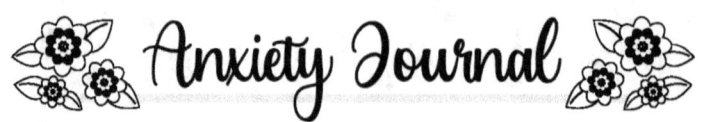

DATE .... TIME ....
PLACE .... SOURCE OF ANXIETY ....
PHYSICAL SENSATIONS ....

NEGATIVE BELIEVES

ABOUT SITUATION ....
....
ABOUT YOUSELF ....
....

WHAT FACTS DO YOU KNOW ARE TRUE?

ABOUT SITUATION ....
....
ABOUT YOUSELF ....
....

WHAT HAPPENED?

....
....

HOW DID IT MAKE YOU FEEL?

....
....

HOW DID YOU REACT?

....
....

WHAT HELPS YOU SOOTHE YOUR ANXIETY?

....
....

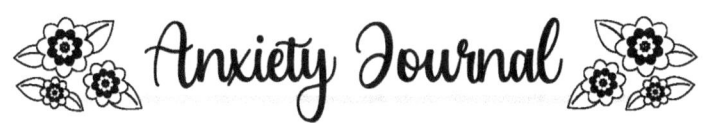

DATE   TIME

PLACE   SOURCE OF ANXIETY

PHYSICAL SENSATIONS

NEGATIVE BELIEVES

ABOUT SITUATION ....
....

ABOUT YOUSELF ....
....

WHAT FACTS DO YOU KNOW ARE TRUE?

ABOUT SITUATION ....
....

ABOUT YOUSELF ....
....

WHAT HAPPENED?

....
....

HOW DID IT MAKE YOU FEEL?

....
....

HOW DID YOU REACT?

....
....

WHAT HELPS YOU SOOTHE YOUR ANXIETY?

....
....

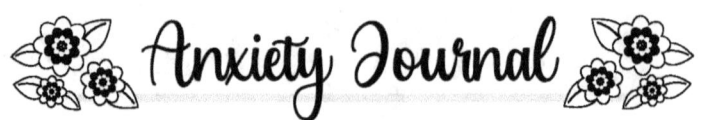

Anxiety Journal

DATE .... **TIME** ....

PLACE .... **SOURCE OF ANXIETY** ....

PHYSICAL SENSATIONS ....

NEGATIVE BELIEVES

ABOUT SITUATION ....
....

ABOUT YOUSELF ....
....

WHAT FACTS DO YOU KNOW ARE TRUE?

ABOUT SITUATION ....
....

ABOUT YOUSELF ....
....

WHAT HAPPENED?

....
....

HOW DID IT MAKE YOU FEEL?

....
....

HOW DID YOU REACT?

....
....

WHAT HELPS YOU SOOTHE YOUR ANXIETY?

....
....

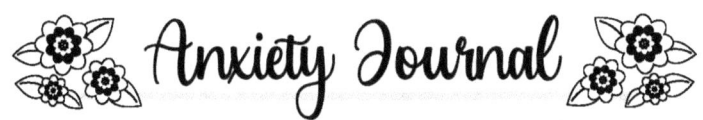

Anxiety Journal

DATE   TIME

PLACE   SOURCE OF ANXIETY

PHYSICAL SENSATIONS

NEGATIVE BELIEVES

ABOUT SITUATION ....

....

ABOUT YOUSELF ....

....

WHAT FACTS DO YOU KNOW ARE TRUE?

ABOUT SITUATION ....

....

ABOUT YOUSELF ....

....

WHAT HAPPENED?

....

....

HOW DID IT MAKE YOU FEEL?

....

....

HOW DID YOU REACT?

....

....

WHAT HELPS YOU SOOTHE YOUR ANXIETY?

....

....

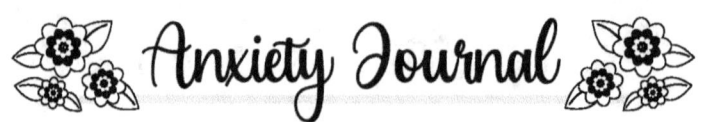

Anxiety Journal

DATE .... **TIME** ....

PLACE .... **SOURCE OF ANXIETY** ....

PHYSICAL SENSATIONS ....

NEGATIVE BELIEVES

ABOUT SITUATION ....
....

ABOUT YOUSELF ....
....

WHAT FACTS DO YOU KNOW ARE TRUE?

ABOUT SITUATION ....
....

ABOUT YOUSELF ....
....

WHAT HAPPENED?

....
....

HOW DID IT MAKE YOU FEEL?

....
....

HOW DID YOU REACT?

....
....

WHAT HELPS YOU SOOTHE YOUR ANXIETY?

....
....

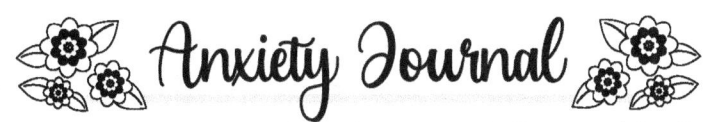
Anxiety Journal

DATE   **TIME**

PLACE   **SOURCE OF ANXIETY**

PHYSICAL SENSATIONS

NEGATIVE BELIEVES

ABOUT SITUATION ....

....

ABOUT YOUSELF ....

....

WHAT FACTS DO YOU KNOW ARE TRUE?

ABOUT SITUATION ....

....

ABOUT YOUSELF ....

....

WHAT HAPPENED?

....

....

HOW DID IT MAKE YOU FEEL?

....

....

HOW DID YOU REACT?

....

....

WHAT HELPS YOU SOOTHE YOUR ANXIETY?

....

....

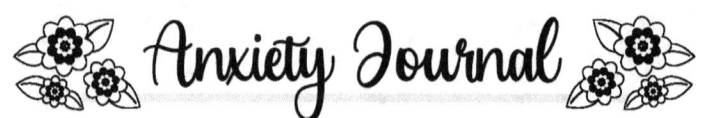

Anxiety Journal

DATE .... **TIME** ....

PLACE .... **SOURCE OF ANXIETY** ....

PHYSICAL SENSATIONS ....

NEGATIVE BELIEVES

ABOUT SITUATION ....
....

ABOUT YOUSELF ....
....

WHAT FACTS DO YOU KNOW ARE TRUE?

ABOUT SITUATION ....
....

ABOUT YOUSELF ....
....

WHAT HAPPENED?

....
....

HOW DID IT MAKE YOU FEEL?

....
....

HOW DID YOU REACT?

....
....

WHAT HELPS YOU SOOTHE YOUR ANXIETY?

....
....

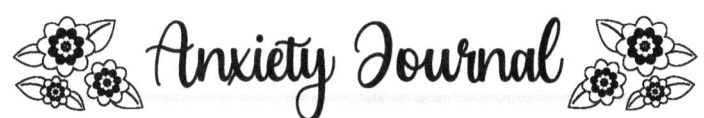

DATE .... **TIME** ....

PLACE .... **SOURCE OF ANXIETY** ....

PHYSICAL SENSATIONS ....

NEGATIVE BELIEVES

ABOUT SITUATION ....
....

ABOUT YOUSELF ....
....

WHAT FACTS DO YOU KNOW ARE TRUE?

ABOUT SITUATION ....
....

ABOUT YOUSELF ....
....

WHAT HAPPENED?

....
....

HOW DID IT MAKE YOU FEEL?

....
....

HOW DID YOU REACT?

....
....

WHAT HELPS YOU SOOTHE YOUR ANXIETY?

....
....

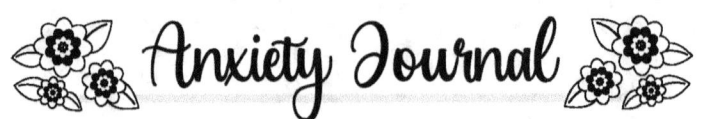

DATE _____ TIME _____

PLACE _____ SOURCE OF ANXIETY _____

PHYSICAL SENSATIONS _____

NEGATIVE BELIEVES

ABOUT SITUATION ....
....

ABOUT YOUSELF ....
....

WHAT FACTS DO YOU KNOW ARE TRUE?

ABOUT SITUATION ....
....

ABOUT YOUSELF ....
....

WHAT HAPPENED?

....
....

HOW DID IT MAKE YOU FEEL?

....
....

HOW DID YOU REACT?

....
....

WHAT HELPS YOU SOOTHE YOUR ANXIETY?

....
....

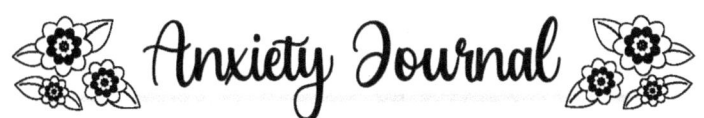

DATE   TIME

PLACE   SOURCE OF ANXIETY

PHYSICAL SENSATIONS

NEGATIVE BELIEVES

ABOUT SITUATION ....
....

ABOUT YOUSELF ....
....

WHAT FACTS DO YOU KNOW ARE TRUE?

ABOUT SITUATION ....
....

ABOUT YOUSELF ....
....

WHAT HAPPENED?

....
....

HOW DID IT MAKE YOU FEEL?

....
....

HOW DID YOU REACT?

....
....

WHAT HELPS YOU SOOTHE YOUR ANXIETY?

....
....

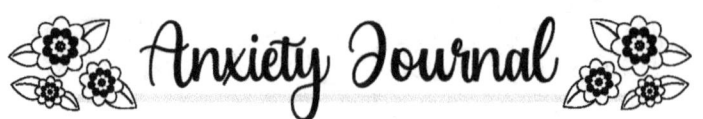

Anxiety Journal

DATE _____ **TIME** _____

PLACE _____ **SOURCE OF ANXIETY** _____

PHYSICAL SENSATIONS _____

NEGATIVE BELIEVES

ABOUT SITUATION ....
....

ABOUT YOUSELF ....
....

WHAT FACTS DO YOU KNOW ARE TRUE?

ABOUT SITUATION ....
....

ABOUT YOUSELF ....
....

WHAT HAPPENED?

....
....

HOW DID IT MAKE YOU FEEL?

....
....

HOW DID YOU REACT?

....
....

WHAT HELPS YOU SOOTHE YOUR ANXIETY?

....
....

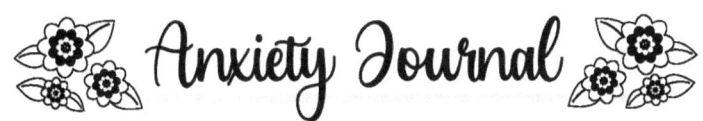

DATE   TIME

PLACE   SOURCE OF ANXIETY

PHYSICAL SENSATIONS

NEGATIVE BELIEVES

ABOUT SITUATION ....
....

ABOUT YOUSELF ....
....

WHAT FACTS DO YOU KNOW ARE TRUE?

ABOUT SITUATION ....
....

ABOUT YOUSELF ....
....

WHAT HAPPENED?

....
....

HOW DID IT MAKE YOU FEEL?

....
....

HOW DID YOU REACT?

....
....

WHAT HELPS YOU SOOTHE YOUR ANXIETY?

....
....

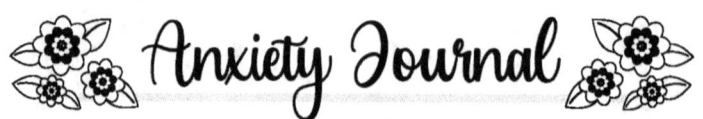

Anxiety Journal

DATE .... TIME ....

PLACE .... SOURCE OF ANXIETY ....

PHYSICAL SENSATIONS ....

NEGATIVE BELIEVES

ABOUT SITUATION ....
....

ABOUT YOUSELF ....
....

WHAT FACTS DO YOU KNOW ARE TRUE?

ABOUT SITUATION ....
....

ABOUT YOUSELF ....
....

WHAT HAPPENED?

....
....

HOW DID IT MAKE YOU FEEL?

....
....

HOW DID YOU REACT?

....
....

WHAT HELPS YOU SOOTHE YOUR ANXIETY?

....
....

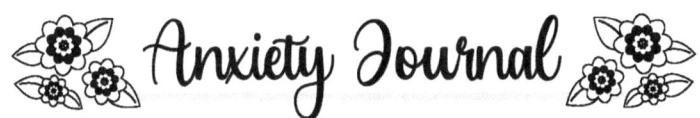

DATE **TIME**

PLACE **SOURCE OF ANXIETY**

PHYSICAL SENSATIONS

NEGATIVE BELIEVES

ABOUT SITUATION ....
....

ABOUT YOUSELF ....
....

WHAT FACTS DO YOU KNOW ARE TRUE?

ABOUT SITUATION ....
....

ABOUT YOUSELF ....
....

WHAT HAPPENED?

....
....

HOW DID IT MAKE YOU FEEL?

....
....

HOW DID YOU REACT?

....
....

WHAT HELPS YOU SOOTHE YOUR ANXIETY?

....
....

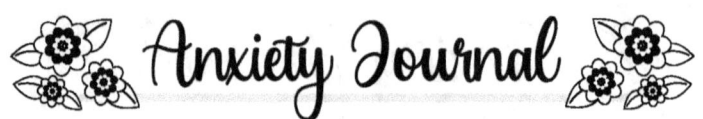
Anxiety Journal

DATE .... **TIME** ....

PLACE .... **SOURCE OF ANXIETY** ....

PHYSICAL SENSATIONS ....

NEGATIVE BELIEVES

ABOUT SITUATION ....
....

ABOUT YOUSELF ....
....

WHAT FACTS DO YOU KNOW ARE TRUE?

ABOUT SITUATION ....
....

ABOUT YOUSELF ....
....

WHAT HAPPENED?
....
....

HOW DID IT MAKE YOU FEEL?
....
....

HOW DID YOU REACT?
....
....

WHAT HELPS YOU SOOTHE YOUR ANXIETY?
....
....

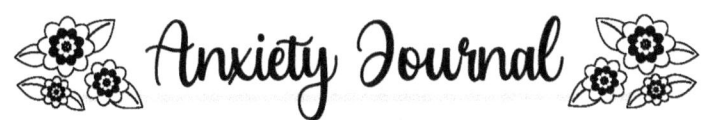

Anxiety Journal

DATE TIME

PLACE SOURCE OF ANXIETY

PHYSICAL SENSATIONS

NEGATIVE BELIEVES

ABOUT SITUATION ....
....

ABOUT YOUSELF ....
....

WHAT FACTS DO YOU KNOW ARE TRUE?

ABOUT SITUATION ....
....

ABOUT YOUSELF ....
....

WHAT HAPPENED?

....
....

HOW DID IT MAKE YOU FEEL?

....
....

HOW DID YOU REACT?

....
....

WHAT HELPS YOU SOOTHE YOUR ANXIETY?

....
....

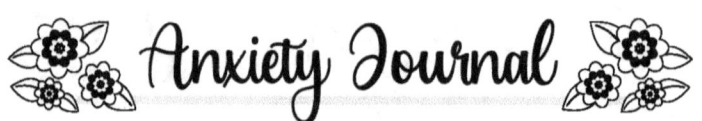

Anxiety Journal

DATE .... TIME ....

PLACE .... SOURCE OF ANXIETY ....

PHYSICAL SENSATIONS ....

NEGATIVE BELIEVES

ABOUT SITUATION ....
....

ABOUT YOUSELF ....
....

WHAT FACTS DO YOU KNOW ARE TRUE?

ABOUT SITUATION ....
....

ABOUT YOUSELF ....
....

WHAT HAPPENED?

....
....

HOW DID IT MAKE YOU FEEL?

....
....

HOW DID YOU REACT?

....
....

WHAT HELPS YOU SOOTHE YOUR ANXIETY?

....
....

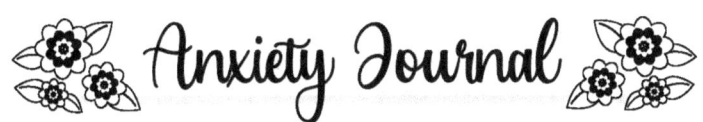

Anxiety Journal

DATE TIME

PLACE SOURCE OF ANXIETY

PHYSICAL SENSATIONS

NEGATIVE BELIEVES

ABOUT SITUATION ....
....

ABOUT YOUSELF ....
....

WHAT FACTS DO YOU KNOW ARE TRUE?

ABOUT SITUATION ....
....

ABOUT YOUSELF ....
....

WHAT HAPPENED?

....
....

HOW DID IT MAKE YOU FEEL?

....
....

HOW DID YOU REACT?

....
....

WHAT HELPS YOU SOOTHE YOUR ANXIETY?

....
....

Anxiety Journal

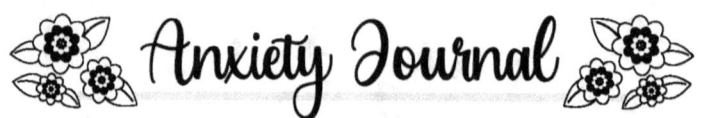

DATE .... TIME ....

PLACE .... SOURCE OF ANXIETY ....

PHYSICAL SENSATIONS ....

NEGATIVE BELIEVES

ABOUT SITUATION ....
....

ABOUT YOUSELF ....
....

WHAT FACTS DO YOU KNOW ARE TRUE?

ABOUT SITUATION ....
....

ABOUT YOUSELF ....
....

WHAT HAPPENED?

....
....

HOW DID IT MAKE YOU FEEL?

....
....

HOW DID YOU REACT?

....
....

WHAT HELPS YOU SOOTHE YOUR ANXIETY?

....
....

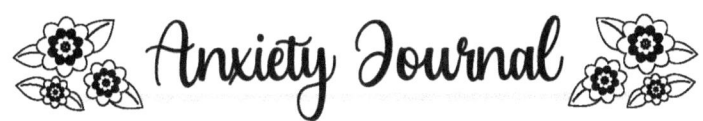

DATE   TIME

PLACE   SOURCE OF ANXIETY

PHYSICAL SENSATIONS

NEGATIVE BELIEVES

ABOUT SITUATION ....

ABOUT YOUSELF ....

WHAT FACTS DO YOU KNOW ARE TRUE?

ABOUT SITUATION ....

ABOUT YOUSELF ....

WHAT HAPPENED?

....
....

HOW DID IT MAKE YOU FEEL?

....
....

HOW DID YOU REACT?

....
....

WHAT HELPS YOU SOOTHE YOUR ANXIETY?

....
....

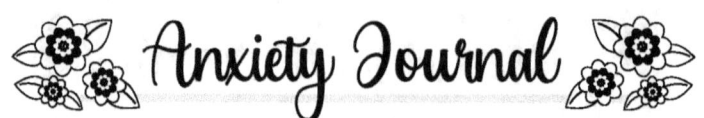

Anxiety Journal

DATE .... **TIME** ....

PLACE .... **SOURCE OF ANXIETY** ....

PHYSICAL SENSATIONS ....

NEGATIVE BELIEVES

ABOUT SITUATION ....
....

ABOUT YOUSELF ....
....

WHAT FACTS DO YOU KNOW ARE TRUE?

ABOUT SITUATION ....
....

ABOUT YOUSELF ....
....

WHAT HAPPENED?

....
....

HOW DID IT MAKE YOU FEEL?

....
....

HOW DID YOU REACT?

....
....

WHAT HELPS YOU SOOTHE YOUR ANXIETY?

....
....

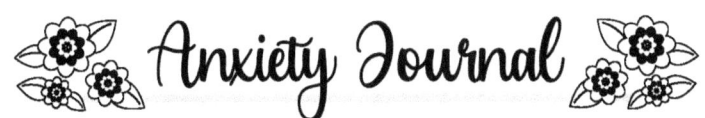

Anxiety Journal

DATE TIME

PLACE SOURCE OF ANXIETY

PHYSICAL SENSATIONS

NEGATIVE BELIEVES

ABOUT SITUATION ....
....

ABOUT YOUSELF ....
....

WHAT FACTS DO YOU KNOW ARE TRUE?

ABOUT SITUATION ....
....

ABOUT YOUSELF ....
....

WHAT HAPPENED?

....
....

HOW DID IT MAKE YOU FEEL?

....
....

HOW DID YOU REACT?

....
....

WHAT HELPS YOU SOOTHE YOUR ANXIETY?

....
....

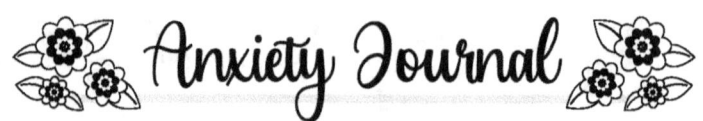

Anxiety Journal

DATE   **TIME**

PLACE   **SOURCE OF ANXIETY**

PHYSICAL SENSATIONS

NEGATIVE BELIEVES

ABOUT SITUATION ....
....

ABOUT YOUSELF ....
....

WHAT FACTS DO YOU KNOW ARE TRUE?

ABOUT SITUATION ....
....

ABOUT YOUSELF ....
....

WHAT HAPPENED?

....
....

HOW DID IT MAKE YOU FEEL?

....
....

HOW DID YOU REACT?

....
....

WHAT HELPS YOU SOOTHE YOUR ANXIETY?

....
....

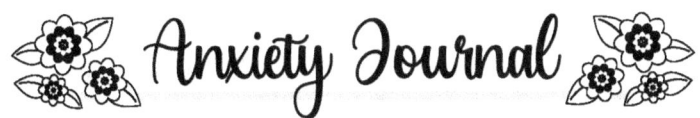

Anxiety Journal

DATE　　　　　　　　　　**TIME**

PLACE　　　　　　　　　**SOURCE OF ANXIETY**

PHYSICAL SENSATIONS

NEGATIVE BELIEVES

ABOUT SITUATION ....
....

ABOUT YOUSELF ....
....

WHAT FACTS DO YOU KNOW ARE TRUE?

ABOUT SITUATION ....
....

ABOUT YOUSELF ....
....

WHAT HAPPENED?

....
....

HOW DID IT MAKE YOU FEEL?

....
....

HOW DID YOU REACT?

....
....

WHAT HELPS YOU SOOTHE YOUR ANXIETY?

....
....

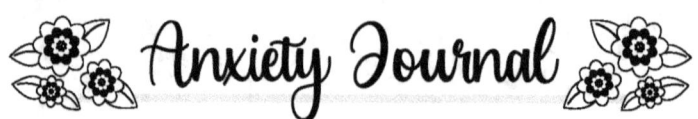

DATE .... TIME ....
PLACE .... SOURCE OF ANXIETY ....
PHYSICAL SENSATIONS ....

NEGATIVE BELIEVES

ABOUT SITUATION ....
....

ABOUT YOUSELF ....
....

WHAT FACTS DO YOU KNOW ARE TRUE?

ABOUT SITUATION ....
....

ABOUT YOUSELF ....
....

WHAT HAPPENED?

....
....

HOW DID IT MAKE YOU FEEL?

....
....

HOW DID YOU REACT?

....
....

WHAT HELPS YOU SOOTHE YOUR ANXIETY?

....
....

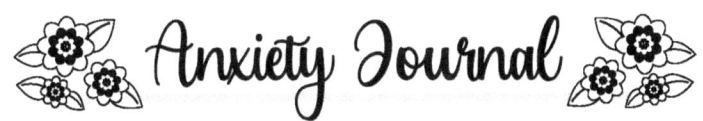

Anxiety Journal

DATE **TIME**

PLACE **SOURCE OF ANXIETY**

PHYSICAL SENSATIONS

NEGATIVE BELIEVES

ABOUT SITUATION ....
....

ABOUT YOUSELF ....
....

WHAT FACTS DO YOU KNOW ARE TRUE?

ABOUT SITUATION ....
....

ABOUT YOUSELF ....
....

WHAT HAPPENED?

....
....

HOW DID IT MAKE YOU FEEL?

....
....

HOW DID YOU REACT?

....
....

WHAT HELPS YOU SOOTHE YOUR ANXIETY?

....
....

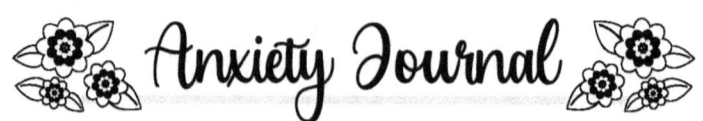
Anxiety Journal

DATE .... TIME ....
PLACE .... SOURCE OF ANXIETY ....
PHYSICAL SENSATIONS ....

NEGATIVE BELIEVES
ABOUT SITUATION ....
....
ABOUT YOUSELF ....
....

WHAT FACTS DO YOU KNOW ARE TRUE?
ABOUT SITUATION ....
....
ABOUT YOUSELF ....
....

WHAT HAPPENED?
....
....

HOW DID IT MAKE YOU FEEL?
....
....

HOW DID YOU REACT?
....
....

WHAT HELPS YOU SOOTHE YOUR ANXIETY?
....
....

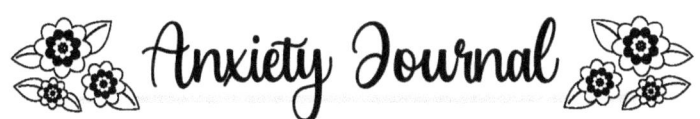

DATE TIME

PLACE SOURCE OF ANXIETY

PHYSICAL SENSATIONS

NEGATIVE BELIEVES

ABOUT SITUATION ....
....

ABOUT YOUSELF ....
....

WHAT FACTS DO YOU KNOW ARE TRUE?

ABOUT SITUATION ....
....

ABOUT YOUSELF ....
....

WHAT HAPPENED?

....
....

HOW DID IT MAKE YOU FEEL?

....
....

HOW DID YOU REACT?

....
....

WHAT HELPS YOU SOOTHE YOUR ANXIETY?

....
....

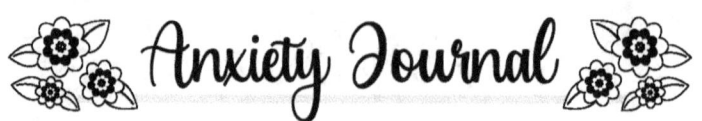

Anxiety Journal

DATE .... TIME ....

PLACE .... SOURCE OF ANXIETY ....

PHYSICAL SENSATIONS ....

NEGATIVE BELIEVES

ABOUT SITUATION ....
....

ABOUT YOUSELF ....
....

WHAT FACTS DO YOU KNOW ARE TRUE?

ABOUT SITUATION ....
....

ABOUT YOUSELF ....
....

WHAT HAPPENED?

....
....

HOW DID IT MAKE YOU FEEL?

....
....

HOW DID YOU REACT?

....
....

WHAT HELPS YOU SOOTHE YOUR ANXIETY?

....
....

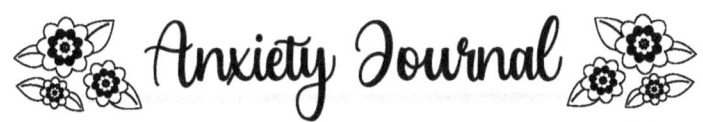

Anxiety Journal

DATE   TIME

PLACE   SOURCE OF ANXIETY

PHYSICAL SENSATIONS

NEGATIVE BELIEVES

ABOUT SITUATION ....

ABOUT YOUSELF ....

WHAT FACTS DO YOU KNOW ARE TRUE?

ABOUT SITUATION ....

ABOUT YOUSELF ....

WHAT HAPPENED?

....

....

HOW DID IT MAKE YOU FEEL?

....

....

HOW DID YOU REACT?

....

....

WHAT HELPS YOU SOOTHE YOUR ANXIETY?

....

....

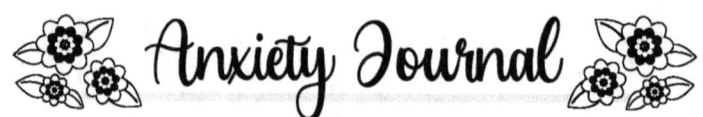

Anxiety Journal

DATE .... **TIME** ....

PLACE .... **SOURCE OF ANXIETY** ....

PHYSICAL SENSATIONS ....

NEGATIVE BELIEVES

ABOUT SITUATION ....
....

ABOUT YOUSELF ....
....

WHAT FACTS DO YOU KNOW ARE TRUE?

ABOUT SITUATION ....
....

ABOUT YOUSELF ....
....

WHAT HAPPENED?

....
....

HOW DID IT MAKE YOU FEEL?

....
....

HOW DID YOU REACT?

....
....

WHAT HELPS YOU SOOTHE YOUR ANXIETY?

....
....

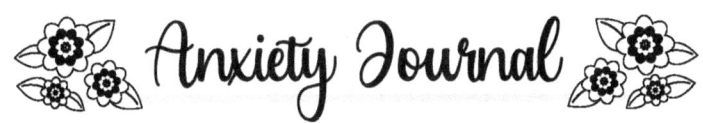

Anxiety Journal

DATE   **TIME**

PLACE   **SOURCE OF ANXIETY**

PHYSICAL SENSATIONS

NEGATIVE BELIEVES

ABOUT SITUATION ....
....

ABOUT YOUSELF ....
....

WHAT FACTS DO YOU KNOW ARE TRUE?

ABOUT SITUATION ....
....

ABOUT YOUSELF ....
....

WHAT HAPPENED?

....
....

HOW DID IT MAKE YOU FEEL?

....
....

HOW DID YOU REACT?

....
....

WHAT HELPS YOU SOOTHE YOUR ANXIETY?

....
....

Anxiety Journal

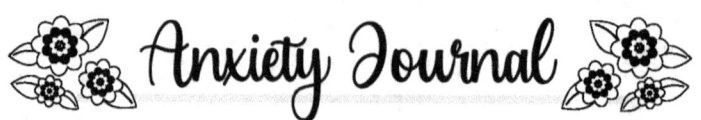

DATE .... **TIME** ....

PLACE .... **SOURCE OF ANXIETY** ....

PHYSICAL SENSATIONS ....

NEGATIVE BELIEVES

ABOUT SITUATION ....
....

ABOUT YOUSELF ....
....

WHAT FACTS DO YOU KNOW ARE TRUE?

ABOUT SITUATION ....
....

ABOUT YOUSELF ....
....

WHAT HAPPENED?

....
....

HOW DID IT MAKE YOU FEEL?

....
....

HOW DID YOU REACT?

....
....

WHAT HELPS YOU SOOTHE YOUR ANXIETY?

....
....

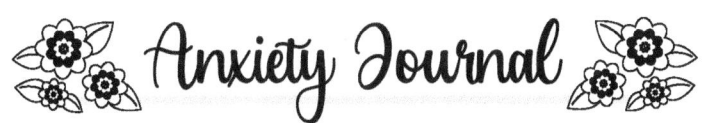

Anxiety Journal

DATE .... **TIME** ....

PLACE .... **SOURCE OF ANXIETY** ....

PHYSICAL SENSATIONS ....

NEGATIVE BELIEVES

ABOUT SITUATION ....
....

ABOUT YOUSELF ....
....

WHAT FACTS DO YOU KNOW ARE TRUE?

ABOUT SITUATION ....
....

ABOUT YOUSELF ....
....

WHAT HAPPENED?

....
....

HOW DID IT MAKE YOU FEEL?

....
....

HOW DID YOU REACT?

....
....

WHAT HELPS YOU SOOTHE YOUR ANXIETY?

....
....

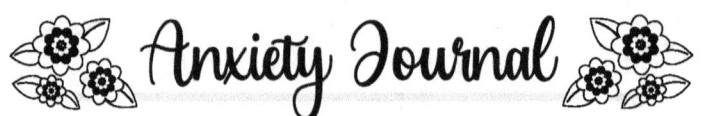

Anxiety Journal

DATE .... **TIME** ....

PLACE .... **SOURCE OF ANXIETY** ....

PHYSICAL SENSATIONS ....

NEGATIVE BELIEVES

ABOUT SITUATION ....
....

ABOUT YOUSELF ....
....

WHAT FACTS DO YOU KNOW ARE TRUE?

ABOUT SITUATION ....
....

ABOUT YOUSELF ....
....

WHAT HAPPENED?

....
....

HOW DID IT MAKE YOU FEEL?

....
....

HOW DID YOU REACT?

....
....

WHAT HELPS YOU SOOTHE YOUR ANXIETY?

....
....

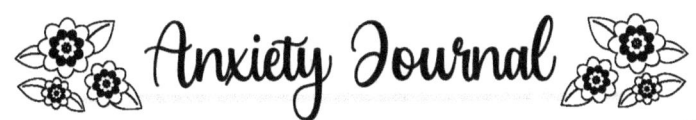

Anxiety Journal

DATE   TIME

PLACE   SOURCE OF ANXIETY

PHYSICAL SENSATIONS

NEGATIVE BELIEVES

ABOUT SITUATION ....

....

ABOUT YOUSELF ....

....

WHAT FACTS DO YOU KNOW ARE TRUE?

ABOUT SITUATION ....

....

ABOUT YOUSELF ....

....

WHAT HAPPENED?

....

....

HOW DID IT MAKE YOU FEEL?

....

....

HOW DID YOU REACT?

....

....

WHAT HELPS YOU SOOTHE YOUR ANXIETY?

....

....

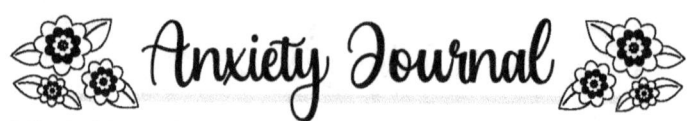

Anxiety Journal

DATE .... **TIME** ....

PLACE .... **SOURCE OF ANXIETY** ....

PHYSICAL SENSATIONS ....

NEGATIVE BELIEVES

ABOUT SITUATION ....
....

ABOUT YOUSELF ....
....

WHAT FACTS DO YOU KNOW ARE TRUE?

ABOUT SITUATION ....
....

ABOUT YOUSELF ....
....

WHAT HAPPENED?

....
....

HOW DID IT MAKE YOU FEEL?

....
....

HOW DID YOU REACT?

....
....

WHAT HELPS YOU SOOTHE YOUR ANXIETY?

....
....

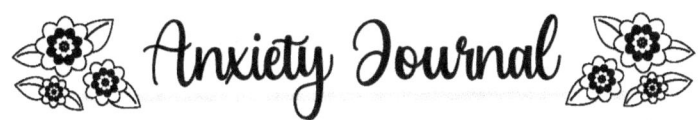

Anxiety Journal

DATE   TIME

PLACE   SOURCE OF ANXIETY

PHYSICAL SENSATIONS

NEGATIVE BELIEVES

ABOUT SITUATION ....
....

ABOUT YOUSELF ....
....

WHAT FACTS DO YOU KNOW ARE TRUE?

ABOUT SITUATION ....
....

ABOUT YOUSELF ....
....

WHAT HAPPENED?

....
....

HOW DID IT MAKE YOU FEEL?

....
....

HOW DID YOU REACT?

....
....

WHAT HELPS YOU SOOTHE YOUR ANXIETY?

....
....

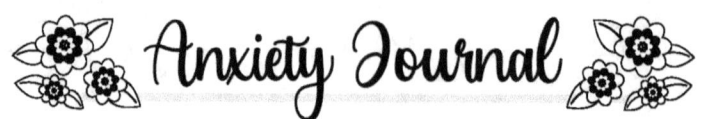

Anxiety Journal

DATE .... TIME ....

PLACE .... SOURCE OF ANXIETY ....

PHYSICAL SENSATIONS ....

NEGATIVE BELIEVES

ABOUT SITUATION ....
....

ABOUT YOUSELF ....
....

WHAT FACTS DO YOU KNOW ARE TRUE?

ABOUT SITUATION ....
....

ABOUT YOUSELF ....
....

WHAT HAPPENED?

....
....

HOW DID IT MAKE YOU FEEL?

....
....

HOW DID YOU REACT?

....
....

WHAT HELPS YOU SOOTHE YOUR ANXIETY?

....
....

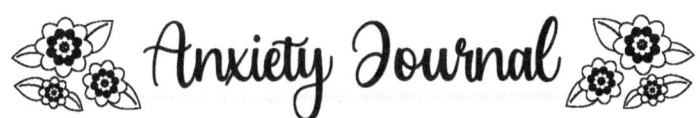

DATE   TIME

PLACE   SOURCE OF ANXIETY

PHYSICAL SENSATIONS

NEGATIVE BELIEVES

ABOUT SITUATION ....
....

ABOUT YOUSELF ....
....

WHAT FACTS DO YOU KNOW ARE TRUE?

ABOUT SITUATION ....
....

ABOUT YOUSELF ....
....

WHAT HAPPENED?

....
....

HOW DID IT MAKE YOU FEEL?

....
....

HOW DID YOU REACT?

....
....

WHAT HELPS YOU SOOTHE YOUR ANXIETY?

....
....

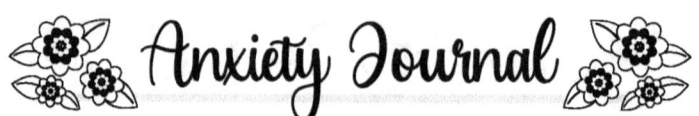

Anxiety Journal

DATE .... **TIME** ....

PLACE .... **SOURCE OF ANXIETY** ....

PHYSICAL SENSATIONS ....

NEGATIVE BELIEVES

ABOUT SITUATION ....
....

ABOUT YOUSELF ....
....

WHAT FACTS DO YOU KNOW ARE TRUE?

ABOUT SITUATION ....
....

ABOUT YOUSELF ....
....

WHAT HAPPENED?

....
....

HOW DID IT MAKE YOU FEEL?

....
....

HOW DID YOU REACT?

....
....

WHAT HELPS YOU SOOTHE YOUR ANXIETY?

....
....

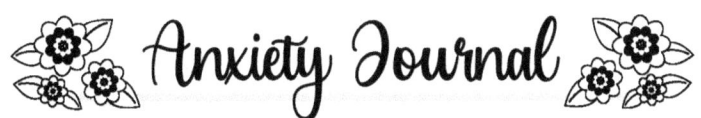

DATE TIME

PLACE SOURCE OF ANXIETY

PHYSICAL SENSATIONS

NEGATIVE BELIEVES

ABOUT SITUATION ....

....

ABOUT YOUSELF ....

....

WHAT FACTS DO YOU KNOW ARE TRUE?

ABOUT SITUATION ....

....

ABOUT YOUSELF ....

....

WHAT HAPPENED?

....

....

HOW DID IT MAKE YOU FEEL?

....

....

HOW DID YOU REACT?

....

....

WHAT HELPS YOU SOOTHE YOUR ANXIETY?

....

....

Anxiety Journal

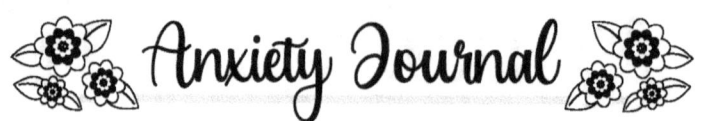

DATE .... **TIME** ....

PLACE .... **SOURCE OF ANXIETY** ....

PHYSICAL SENSATIONS ....

NEGATIVE BELIEVES

ABOUT SITUATION ....
....

ABOUT YOUSELF ....
....

WHAT FACTS DO YOU KNOW ARE TRUE?

ABOUT SITUATION ....
....

ABOUT YOUSELF ....
....

WHAT HAPPENED?

....
....

HOW DID IT MAKE YOU FEEL?

....
....

HOW DID YOU REACT?

....
....

WHAT HELPS YOU SOOTHE YOUR ANXIETY?

....
....

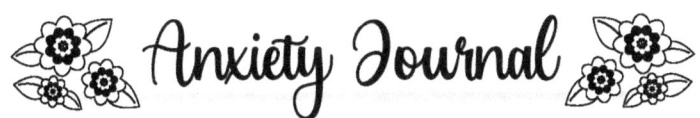

Anxiety Journal

DATE   TIME

PLACE   SOURCE OF ANXIETY

PHYSICAL SENSATIONS

NEGATIVE BELIEVES

ABOUT SITUATION ....
....

ABOUT YOUSELF ....
....

WHAT FACTS DO YOU KNOW ARE TRUE?

ABOUT SITUATION ....
....

ABOUT YOUSELF ....
....

WHAT HAPPENED?

....
....

HOW DID IT MAKE YOU FEEL?

....
....

HOW DID YOU REACT?

....
....

WHAT HELPS YOU SOOTHE YOUR ANXIETY?

....
....

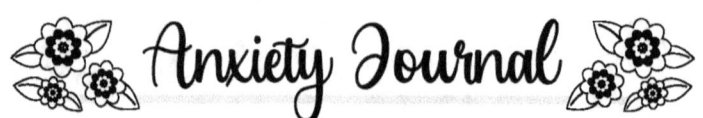

DATE .... TIME ....
PLACE .... SOURCE OF ANXIETY ....
PHYSICAL SENSATIONS ....

NEGATIVE BELIEVES

ABOUT SITUATION ....
....

ABOUT YOUSELF ....
....

WHAT FACTS DO YOU KNOW ARE TRUE?

ABOUT SITUATION ....
....

ABOUT YOUSELF ....
....

WHAT HAPPENED?

....
....

HOW DID IT MAKE YOU FEEL?

....
....

HOW DID YOU REACT?

....
....

WHAT HELPS YOU SOOTHE YOUR ANXIETY?

....
....

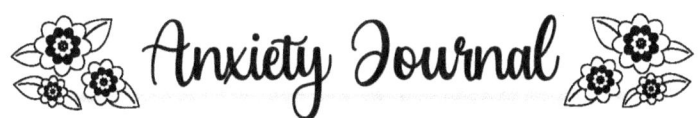

Anxiety Journal

DATE   TIME

PLACE   SOURCE OF ANXIETY

PHYSICAL SENSATIONS

NEGATIVE BELIEVES

ABOUT SITUATION ....
....

ABOUT YOUSELF ....
....

WHAT FACTS DO YOU KNOW ARE TRUE?

ABOUT SITUATION ....
....

ABOUT YOUSELF ....
....

WHAT HAPPENED?

....
....

HOW DID IT MAKE YOU FEEL?

....
....

HOW DID YOU REACT?

....
....

WHAT HELPS YOU SOOTHE YOUR ANXIETY?

....
....

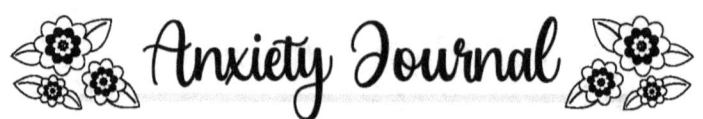

Anxiety Journal

DATE .... **TIME** ....

PLACE .... **SOURCE OF ANXIETY** ....

PHYSICAL SENSATIONS ....

NEGATIVE BELIEVES

ABOUT SITUATION ....
....

ABOUT YOUSELF ....
....

WHAT FACTS DO YOU KNOW ARE TRUE?

ABOUT SITUATION ....
....

ABOUT YOUSELF ....
....

WHAT HAPPENED?

....
....

HOW DID IT MAKE YOU FEEL?

....
....

HOW DID YOU REACT?

....
....

WHAT HELPS YOU SOOTHE YOUR ANXIETY?

....
....

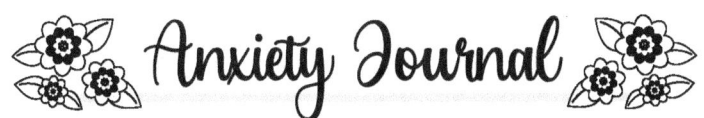

DATE TIME

PLACE SOURCE OF ANXIETY

PHYSICAL SENSATIONS

NEGATIVE BELIEVES

ABOUT SITUATION ....
....

ABOUT YOUSELF ....
....

WHAT FACTS DO YOU KNOW ARE TRUE?

ABOUT SITUATION ....
....

ABOUT YOUSELF ....
....

WHAT HAPPENED?

....
....

HOW DID IT MAKE YOU FEEL?

....
....

HOW DID YOU REACT?

....
....

WHAT HELPS YOU SOOTHE YOUR ANXIETY?

....
....

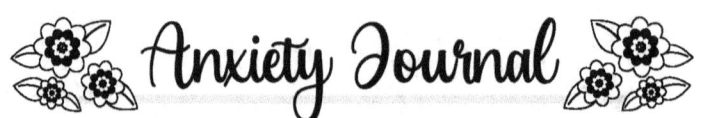

DATE .... TIME ....

PLACE .... SOURCE OF ANXIETY ....

PHYSICAL SENSATIONS ....

NEGATIVE BELIEVES

ABOUT SITUATION ....
....

ABOUT YOURSELF ....
....

WHAT FACTS DO YOU KNOW ARE TRUE?

ABOUT SITUATION ....
....

ABOUT YOUSELF ....
....

WHAT HAPPENED?

....
....

HOW DID IT MAKE YOU FEEL?

....
....

HOW DID YOU REACT?

....
....

WHAT HELPS YOU SOOTHE YOUR ANXIETY?

....
....

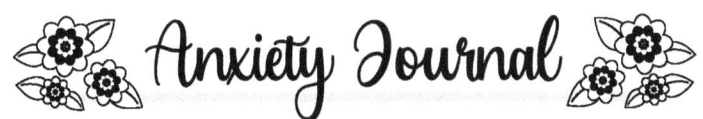

DATE .... TIME ....

PLACE .... SOURCE OF ANXIETY ....

PHYSICAL SENSATIONS ....

NEGATIVE BELIEVES

ABOUT SITUATION ....
....

ABOUT YOUSELF ....
....

WHAT FACTS DO YOU KNOW ARE TRUE?

ABOUT SITUATION ....
....

ABOUT YOUSELF ....
....

WHAT HAPPENED?

....
....

HOW DID IT MAKE YOU FEEL?

....
....

HOW DID YOU REACT?

....
....

WHAT HELPS YOU SOOTHE YOUR ANXIETY?

....
....

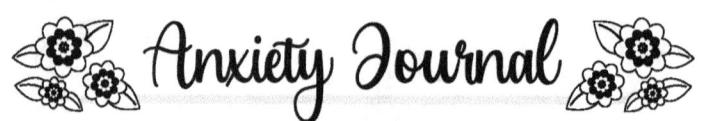

Anxiety Journal

DATE _____ **TIME** _____

PLACE _____ **SOURCE OF ANXIETY** _____

PHYSICAL SENSATIONS _____

NEGATIVE BELIEVES

ABOUT SITUATION ....
....

ABOUT YOUSELF ....
....

WHAT FACTS DO YOU KNOW ARE TRUE?

ABOUT SITUATION ....
....

ABOUT YOUSELF ....
....

WHAT HAPPENED?

....
....

HOW DID IT MAKE YOU FEEL?

....
....

HOW DID YOU REACT?

....
....

WHAT HELPS YOU SOOTHE YOUR ANXIETY?

....
....

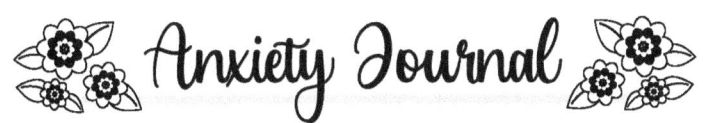

Anxiety Journal

DATE .... TIME ....

PLACE .... SOURCE OF ANXIETY ....

PHYSICAL SENSATIONS ....

NEGATIVE BELIEVES

ABOUT SITUATION ....
....

ABOUT YOUSELF ....
....

WHAT FACTS DO YOU KNOW ARE TRUE?

ABOUT SITUATION ....
....

ABOUT YOUSELF ....
....

WHAT HAPPENED?

....
....

HOW DID IT MAKE YOU FEEL?

....
....

HOW DID YOU REACT?

....
....

WHAT HELPS YOU SOOTHE YOUR ANXIETY?

....
....

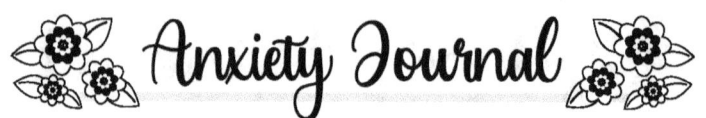

Anxiety Journal

DATE .... TIME ....
PLACE .... SOURCE OF ANXIETY ....
PHYSICAL SENSATIONS ....

NEGATIVE BELIEVES

ABOUT SITUATION ....
....

ABOUT YOUSELF ....
....

WHAT FACTS DO YOU KNOW ARE TRUE?

ABOUT SITUATION ....
....

ABOUT YOUSELF ....
....

WHAT HAPPENED?

....
....

HOW DID IT MAKE YOU FEEL?

....
....

HOW DID YOU REACT?

....
....

WHAT HELPS YOU SOOTHE YOUR ANXIETY?

....
....

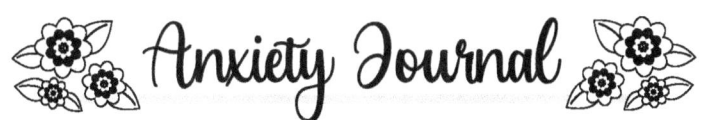

Anxiety Journal

DATE   **TIME**

PLACE   **SOURCE OF ANXIETY**

PHYSICAL SENSATIONS

NEGATIVE BELIEVES

ABOUT SITUATION ....
....

ABOUT YOUSELF ....
....

WHAT FACTS DO YOU KNOW ARE TRUE?

ABOUT SITUATION ....
....

ABOUT YOUSELF ....
....

WHAT HAPPENED?

....
....

HOW DID IT MAKE YOU FEEL?

....
....

HOW DID YOU REACT?

....
....

WHAT HELPS YOU SOOTHE YOUR ANXIETY?

....
....

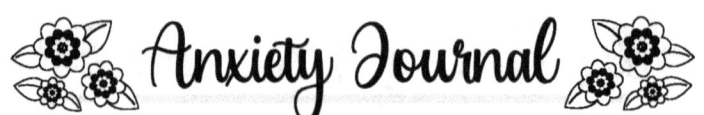

DATE .... TIME ....

PLACE .... SOURCE OF ANXIETY ....

PHYSICAL SENSATIONS ....

NEGATIVE BELIEVES

ABOUT SITUATION ....
....

ABOUT YOUSELF ....
....

WHAT FACTS DO YOU KNOW ARE TRUE?

ABOUT SITUATION ....
....

ABOUT YOUSELF ....
....

WHAT HAPPENED?

....
....

HOW DID IT MAKE YOU FEEL?

....
....

HOW DID YOU REACT?

....
....

WHAT HELPS YOU SOOTHE YOUR ANXIETY?

....
....

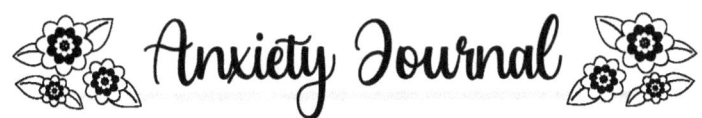

DATE   TIME

PLACE   SOURCE OF ANXIETY

PHYSICAL SENSATIONS

NEGATIVE BELIEVES

ABOUT SITUATION ....
....

ABOUT YOUSELF ....
....

WHAT FACTS DO YOU KNOW ARE TRUE?

ABOUT SITUATION ....
....

ABOUT YOUSELF ....
....

WHAT HAPPENED?

....
....

HOW DID IT MAKE YOU FEEL?

....
....

HOW DID YOU REACT?

....
....

WHAT HELPS YOU SOOTHE YOUR ANXIETY?

....
....

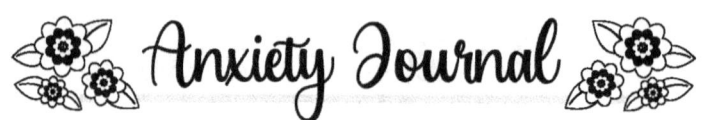
Anxiety Journal

DATE .... TIME ....

PLACE .... SOURCE OF ANXIETY ....

PHYSICAL SENSATIONS ....

NEGATIVE BELIEVES

ABOUT SITUATION ....
....

ABOUT YOUSELF ....
....

WHAT FACTS DO YOU KNOW ARE TRUE?

ABOUT SITUATION ....
....

ABOUT YOUSELF ....
....

WHAT HAPPENED?

....
....

HOW DID IT MAKE YOU FEEL?

....
....

HOW DID YOU REACT?

....
....

WHAT HELPS YOU SOOTHE YOUR ANXIETY?

....
....

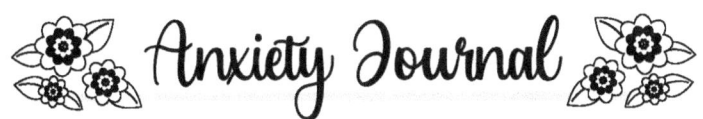

Anxiety Journal

DATE **TIME**

PLACE **SOURCE OF ANXIETY**

PHYSICAL SENSATIONS

NEGATIVE BELIEVES

ABOUT SITUATION ....
....

ABOUT YOUSELF ....
....

WHAT FACTS DO YOU KNOW ARE TRUE?

ABOUT SITUATION ....
....

ABOUT YOUSELF ....
....

WHAT HAPPENED?

....
....

HOW DID IT MAKE YOU FEEL?

....
....

HOW DID YOU REACT?

....
....

WHAT HELPS YOU SOOTHE YOUR ANXIETY?

....
....

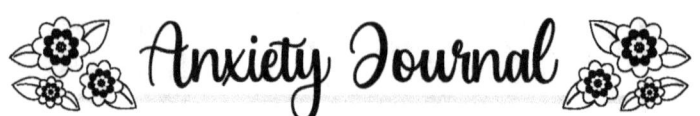

Anxiety Journal

DATE .... TIME ....
PLACE .... SOURCE OF ANXIETY ....
PHYSICAL SENSATIONS ....

NEGATIVE BELIEVES

ABOUT SITUATION ....
....

ABOUT YOUSELF ....
....

WHAT FACTS DO YOU KNOW ARE TRUE?

ABOUT SITUATION ....
....

ABOUT YOUSELF ....
....

WHAT HAPPENED?

....
....

HOW DID IT MAKE YOU FEEL?

....
....

HOW DID YOU REACT?

....
....

WHAT HELPS YOU SOOTHE YOUR ANXIETY?

....
....

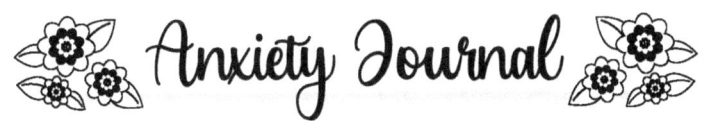

Anxiety Journal

DATE **TIME**

PLACE **SOURCE OF ANXIETY**

PHYSICAL SENSATIONS

NEGATIVE BELIEVES

ABOUT SITUATION ....
....

ABOUT YOUSELF ....
....

WHAT FACTS DO YOU KNOW ARE TRUE?

ABOUT SITUATION ....
....

ABOUT YOUSELF ....
....

WHAT HAPPENED?

....
....

HOW DID IT MAKE YOU FEEL?

....
....

HOW DID YOU REACT?

....
....

WHAT HELPS YOU SOOTHE YOUR ANXIETY?

....
....

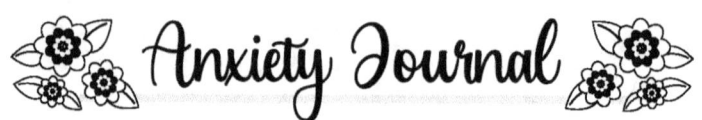

Anxiety Journal

DATE .... TIME ....

PLACE .... SOURCE OF ANXIETY ....

PHYSICAL SENSATIONS ....

NEGATIVE BELIEVES

ABOUT SITUATION ....
....

ABOUT YOUSELF ....
....

WHAT FACTS DO YOU KNOW ARE TRUE?

ABOUT SITUATION ....
....

ABOUT YOUSELF ....
....

WHAT HAPPENED?

....
....

HOW DID IT MAKE YOU FEEL?

....
....

HOW DID YOU REACT?

....
....

WHAT HELPS YOU SOOTHE YOUR ANXIETY?

....
....

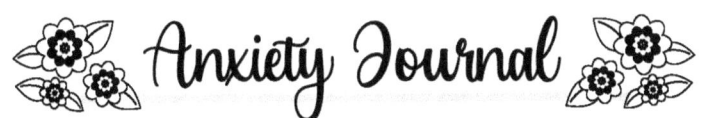

DATE TIME

PLACE SOURCE OF ANXIETY

PHYSICAL SENSATIONS

NEGATIVE BELIEVES

ABOUT SITUATION ....
....

ABOUT YOUSELF ....
....

WHAT FACTS DO YOU KNOW ARE TRUE?

ABOUT SITUATION ....
....

ABOUT YOUSELF ....
....

WHAT HAPPENED?
....
....

HOW DID IT MAKE YOU FEEL?
....
....

HOW DID YOU REACT?
....
....

WHAT HELPS YOU SOOTHE YOUR ANXIETY?
....
....

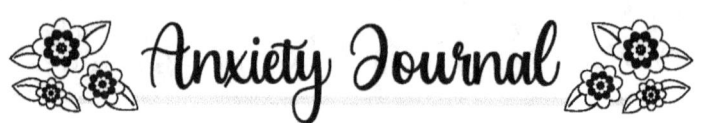

Anxiety Journal

DATE **TIME**

PLACE **SOURCE OF ANXIETY**

PHYSICAL SENSATIONS

NEGATIVE BELIEVES

ABOUT SITUATION ....
....

ABOUT YOUSELF ....
....

WHAT FACTS DO YOU KNOW ARE TRUE?

ABOUT SITUATION ....
....

ABOUT YOUSELF ....
....

WHAT HAPPENED?

....
....

HOW DID IT MAKE YOU FEEL?

....
....

HOW DID YOU REACT?

....
....

WHAT HELPS YOU SOOTHE YOUR ANXIETY?

....
....

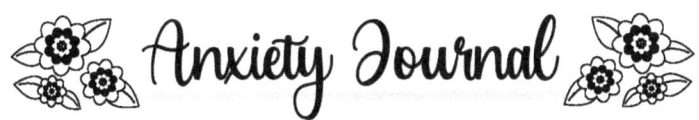

DATE TIME

PLACE SOURCE OF ANXIETY

PHYSICAL SENSATIONS

NEGATIVE BELIEVES

ABOUT SITUATION ....
....

ABOUT YOURSELF ....
....

WHAT FACTS DO YOU KNOW ARE TRUE?

ABOUT SITUATION ....
....

ABOUT YOUSELF ....
....

WHAT HAPPENED?

....
....

HOW DID IT MAKE YOU FEEL?

....
....

HOW DID YOU REACT?

....
....

WHAT HELPS YOU SOOTHE YOUR ANXIETY?

....
....

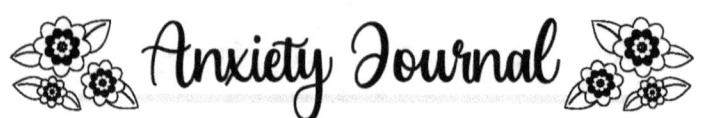

Anxiety Journal

DATE .... TIME ....
PLACE .... SOURCE OF ANXIETY ....
PHYSICAL SENSATIONS ....

NEGATIVE BELIEVES

ABOUT SITUATION ....
....

ABOUT YOUSELF ....
....

WHAT FACTS DO YOU KNOW ARE TRUE?

ABOUT SITUATION ....
....

ABOUT YOUSELF ....
....

WHAT HAPPENED?

....
....

HOW DID IT MAKE YOU FEEL?

....
....

HOW DID YOU REACT?

....
....

WHAT HELPS YOU SOOTHE YOUR ANXIETY?

....
....

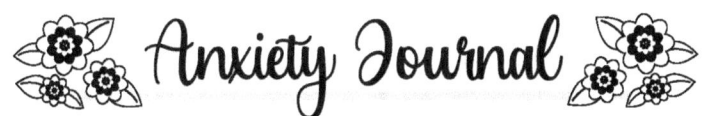

DATE   TIME

PLACE   SOURCE OF ANXIETY

PHYSICAL SENSATIONS

NEGATIVE BELIEVES

ABOUT SITUATION ....
....

ABOUT YOUSELF ....
....

WHAT FACTS DO YOU KNOW ARE TRUE?

ABOUT SITUATION ....
....

ABOUT YOUSELF ....
....

WHAT HAPPENED?

....
....

HOW DID IT MAKE YOU FEEL?

....
....

HOW DID YOU REACT?

....
....

WHAT HELPS YOU SOOTHE YOUR ANXIETY?

....
....

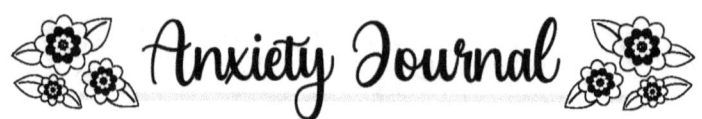
Anxiety Journal

DATE   **TIME**

PLACE   **SOURCE OF ANXIETY**

PHYSICAL SENSATIONS

NEGATIVE BELIEVES

ABOUT SITUATION ....
....

ABOUT YOUSELF ....
....

WHAT FACTS DO YOU KNOW ARE TRUE?

ABOUT SITUATION ....
....

ABOUT YOUSELF ....
....

WHAT HAPPENED?

....
....

HOW DID IT MAKE YOU FEEL?

....
....

HOW DID YOU REACT?

....
....

WHAT HELPS YOU SOOTHE YOUR ANXIETY?

....
....

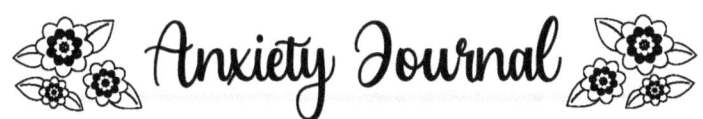

Anxiety Journal

DATE   TIME

PLACE   SOURCE OF ANXIETY

PHYSICAL SENSATIONS

NEGATIVE BELIEVES

ABOUT SITUATION ....
....

ABOUT YOUSELF ....
....

WHAT FACTS DO YOU KNOW ARE TRUE?

ABOUT SITUATION ....
....

ABOUT YOUSELF ....
....

WHAT HAPPENED?

....
....

HOW DID IT MAKE YOU FEEL?

....
....

HOW DID YOU REACT?

....
....

WHAT HELPS YOU SOOTHE YOUR ANXIETY?

....
....

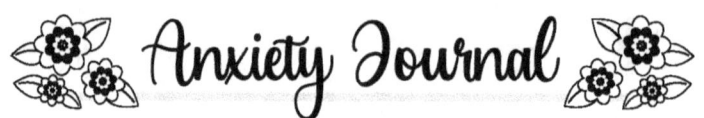

Anxiety Journal

DATE .... TIME ....

PLACE .... SOURCE OF ANXIETY ....

PHYSICAL SENSATIONS ....

NEGATIVE BELIEVES

ABOUT SITUATION ....
....

ABOUT YOUSELF ....
....

WHAT FACTS DO YOU KNOW ARE TRUE?

ABOUT SITUATION ....
....

ABOUT YOUSELF ....
....

WHAT HAPPENED?

....
....

HOW DID IT MAKE YOU FEEL?

....
....

HOW DID YOU REACT?

....
....

WHAT HELPS YOU SOOTHE YOUR ANXIETY?

....
....

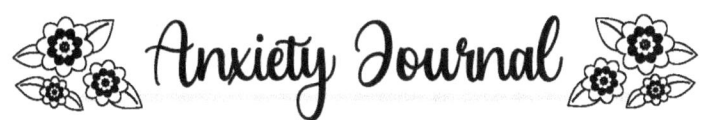

Anxiety Journal

DATE   TIME

PLACE   SOURCE OF ANXIETY

PHYSICAL SENSATIONS

NEGATIVE BELIEVES

ABOUT SITUATION ....

....

ABOUT YOUSELF ....

....

WHAT FACTS DO YOU KNOW ARE TRUE?

ABOUT SITUATION ....

....

ABOUT YOUSELF ....

....

WHAT HAPPENED?

....

....

HOW DID IT MAKE YOU FEEL?

....

....

HOW DID YOU REACT?

....

....

WHAT HELPS YOU SOOTHE YOUR ANXIETY?

....

....

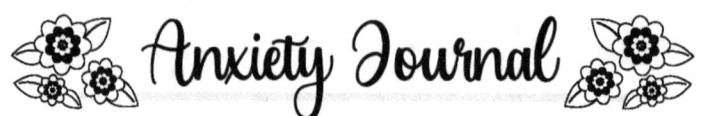

DATE .... TIME ....
PLACE .... SOURCE OF ANXIETY ....
PHYSICAL SENSATIONS ....

NEGATIVE BELIEVES

ABOUT SITUATION ....
....

ABOUT YOUSELF ....
....

WHAT FACTS DO YOU KNOW ARE TRUE?

ABOUT SITUATION ....
....

ABOUT YOUSELF ....
....

WHAT HAPPENED?

....
....

HOW DID IT MAKE YOU FEEL?

....
....

HOW DID YOU REACT?

....
....

WHAT HELPS YOU SOOTHE YOUR ANXIETY?

....
....

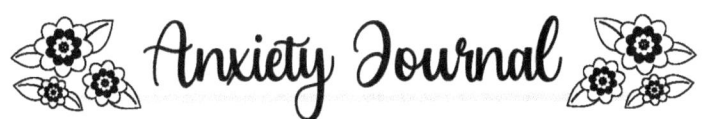

DATE   **TIME**

PLACE   **SOURCE OF ANXIETY**

PHYSICAL SENSATIONS

NEGATIVE BELIEVES

ABOUT SITUATION ....

....

ABOUT YOUSELF ....

....

WHAT FACTS DO YOU KNOW ARE TRUE?

ABOUT SITUATION ....

....

ABOUT YOUSELF ....

....

WHAT HAPPENED?

....

....

HOW DID IT MAKE YOU FEEL?

....

....

HOW DID YOU REACT?

....

....

WHAT HELPS YOU SOOTHE YOUR ANXIETY?

....

....

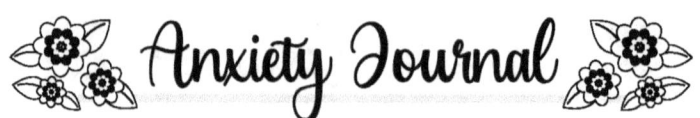

Anxiety Journal

DATE .... TIME ....

PLACE .... SOURCE OF ANXIETY ....

PHYSICAL SENSATIONS ....

NEGATIVE BELIEVES

ABOUT SITUATION ....
....

ABOUT YOUSELF ....
....

WHAT FACTS DO YOU KNOW ARE TRUE?

ABOUT SITUATION ....
....

ABOUT YOUSELF ....
....

WHAT HAPPENED?

....
....

HOW DID IT MAKE YOU FEEL?

....
....

HOW DID YOU REACT?

....
....

WHAT HELPS YOU SOOTHE YOUR ANXIETY?

....
....

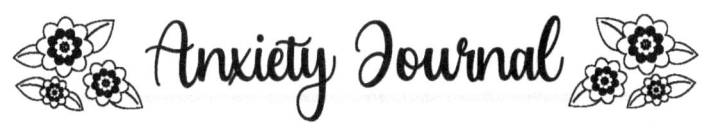

Anxiety Journal

DATE   TIME

PLACE   SOURCE OF ANXIETY

PHYSICAL SENSATIONS

NEGATIVE BELIEVES

ABOUT SITUATION ....
....

ABOUT YOUSELF ....
....

WHAT FACTS DO YOU KNOW ARE TRUE?

ABOUT SITUATION ....
....

ABOUT YOUSELF ....
....

WHAT HAPPENED?

....
....

HOW DID IT MAKE YOU FEEL?

....
....

HOW DID YOU REACT?

....
....

WHAT HELPS YOU SOOTHE YOUR ANXIETY?

....
....

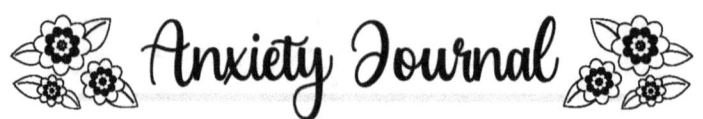

DATE .... TIME ....
PLACE .... SOURCE OF ANXIETY ....
PHYSICAL SENSATIONS ....

NEGATIVE BELIEVES

ABOUT SITUATION ....
....

ABOUT YOUSELF ....
....

WHAT FACTS DO YOU KNOW ARE TRUE?

ABOUT SITUATION ....
....

ABOUT YOUSELF ....
....

WHAT HAPPENED?

....
....

HOW DID IT MAKE YOU FEEL?

....
....

HOW DID YOU REACT?

....
....

WHAT HELPS YOU SOOTHE YOUR ANXIETY?

....
....

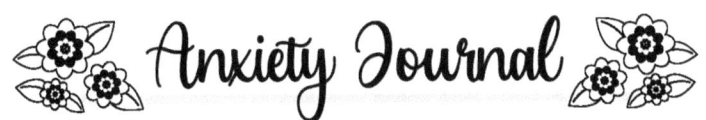

Anxiety Journal

DATE TIME

PLACE SOURCE OF ANXIETY

PHYSICAL SENSATIONS

NEGATIVE BELIEVES

ABOUT SITUATION ....
....

ABOUT YOUSELF ....
....

WHAT FACTS DO YOU KNOW ARE TRUE?

ABOUT SITUATION ....
....

ABOUT YOUSELF ....
....

WHAT HAPPENED?

....
....

HOW DID IT MAKE YOU FEEL?

....
....

HOW DID YOU REACT?

....
....

WHAT HELPS YOU SOOTHE YOUR ANXIETY?

....
....

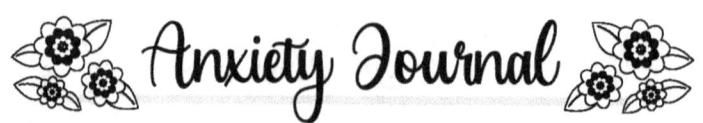

Anxiety Journal

DATE   **TIME**

PLACE   **SOURCE OF ANXIETY**

PHYSICAL SENSATIONS

NEGATIVE BELIEVES

ABOUT SITUATION ....
....

ABOUT YOUSELF ....
....

WHAT FACTS DO YOU KNOW ARE TRUE?

ABOUT SITUATION ....
....

ABOUT YOUSELF ....
....

WHAT HAPPENED?

....
....

HOW DID IT MAKE YOU FEEL?

....
....

HOW DID YOU REACT?

....
....

WHAT HELPS YOU SOOTHE YOUR ANXIETY?

....
....

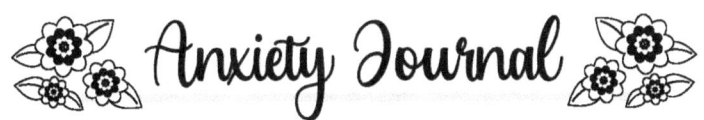

Anxiety Journal

DATE   TIME

PLACE   SOURCE OF ANXIETY

PHYSICAL SENSATIONS

NEGATIVE BELIEVES

ABOUT SITUATION ....
....

ABOUT YOUSELF ....
....

WHAT FACTS DO YOU KNOW ARE TRUE?

ABOUT SITUATION ....
....

ABOUT YOUSELF ....
....

WHAT HAPPENED?

....
....

HOW DID IT MAKE YOU FEEL?

....
....

HOW DID YOU REACT?

....
....

WHAT HELPS YOU SOOTHE YOUR ANXIETY?

....
....

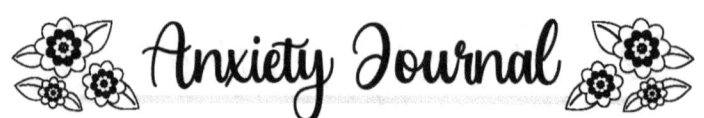

Anxiety Journal

DATE .... TIME ....
PLACE .... SOURCE OF ANXIETY ....
PHYSICAL SENSATIONS ....

NEGATIVE BELIEVES

ABOUT SITUATION ....
....

ABOUT YOUSELF ....
....

WHAT FACTS DO YOU KNOW ARE TRUE?

ABOUT SITUATION ....
....

ABOUT YOUSELF ....
....

WHAT HAPPENED?

....
....

HOW DID IT MAKE YOU FEEL?

....
....

HOW DID YOU REACT?

....
....

WHAT HELPS YOU SOOTHE YOUR ANXIETY?

....
....

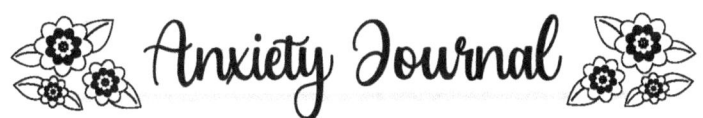
Anxiety Journal

DATE   TIME
PLACE   SOURCE OF ANXIETY
PHYSICAL SENSATIONS

NEGATIVE BELIEVES

ABOUT SITUATION ....
....

ABOUT YOUSELF ....
....

WHAT FACTS DO YOU KNOW ARE TRUE?

ABOUT SITUATION ....
....

ABOUT YOUSELF ....
....

WHAT HAPPENED?

....
....

HOW DID IT MAKE YOU FEEL?

....
....

HOW DID YOU REACT?

....
....

WHAT HELPS YOU SOOTHE YOUR ANXIETY?

....
....

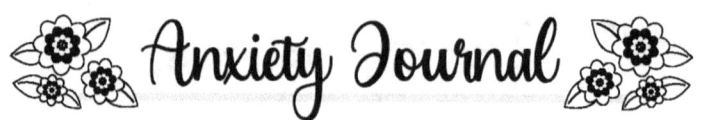

Anxiety Journal

DATE .... **TIME** ....

PLACE .... **SOURCE OF ANXIETY** ....

PHYSICAL SENSATIONS ....

NEGATIVE BELIEVES

ABOUT SITUATION ....
....

ABOUT YOUSELF ....
....

WHAT FACTS DO YOU KNOW ARE TRUE?

ABOUT SITUATION ....
....

ABOUT YOUSELF ....
....

WHAT HAPPENED?

....
....

HOW DID IT MAKE YOU FEEL?

....
....

HOW DID YOU REACT?

....
....

WHAT HELPS YOU SOOTHE YOUR ANXIETY?

....
....

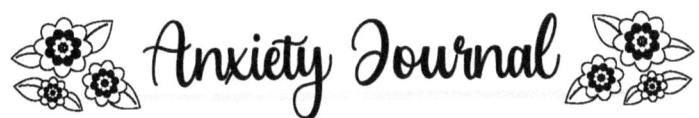

Anxiety Journal

DATE   TIME

PLACE   SOURCE OF ANXIETY

PHYSICAL SENSATIONS

NEGATIVE BELIEVES

ABOUT SITUATION ....

....

ABOUT YOUSELF ....

....

WHAT FACTS DO YOU KNOW ARE TRUE?

ABOUT SITUATION ....

....

ABOUT YOUSELF ....

....

WHAT HAPPENED?

....

....

HOW DID IT MAKE YOU FEEL?

....

....

HOW DID YOU REACT?

....

....

WHAT HELPS YOU SOOTHE YOUR ANXIETY?

....

....

Anxiety Journal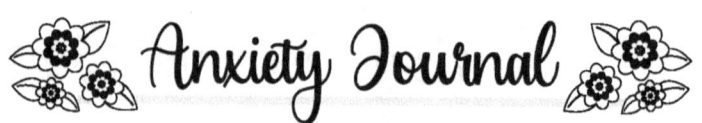

DATE   **TIME**

PLACE   **SOURCE OF ANXIETY**

PHYSICAL SENSATIONS

NEGATIVE BELIEVES

ABOUT SITUATION ....
....

ABOUT YOUSELF ....
....

WHAT FACTS DO YOU KNOW ARE TRUE?

ABOUT SITUATION ....
....

ABOUT YOUSELF ....
....

WHAT HAPPENED?

....
....

HOW DID IT MAKE YOU FEEL?

....
....

HOW DID YOU REACT?

....
....

WHAT HELPS YOU SOOTHE YOUR ANXIETY?

....
....

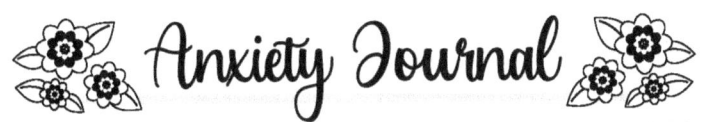

Anxiety Journal

DATE   TIME

PLACE   SOURCE OF ANXIETY

PHYSICAL SENSATIONS

NEGATIVE BELIEVES

ABOUT SITUATION ....
....

ABOUT YOUSELF ....
....

WHAT FACTS DO YOU KNOW ARE TRUE?

ABOUT SITUATION ....
....

ABOUT YOUSELF ....
....

WHAT HAPPENED?

....
....

HOW DID IT MAKE YOU FEEL?

....
....

HOW DID YOU REACT?

....
....

WHAT HELPS YOU SOOTHE YOUR ANXIETY?

....
....

Anxiety Journal

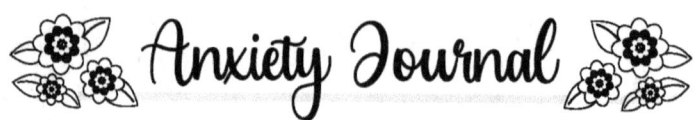

DATE .... **TIME** ....

PLACE .... **SOURCE OF ANXIETY** ....

PHYSICAL SENSATIONS ....

NEGATIVE BELIEVES

ABOUT SITUATION ....
....

ABOUT YOUSELF ....
....

WHAT FACTS DO YOU KNOW ARE TRUE?

ABOUT SITUATION ....
....

ABOUT YOUSELF ....
....

WHAT HAPPENED?

....
....

HOW DID IT MAKE YOU FEEL?

....
....

HOW DID YOU REACT?

....
....

WHAT HELPS YOU SOOTHE YOUR ANXIETY?

....
....

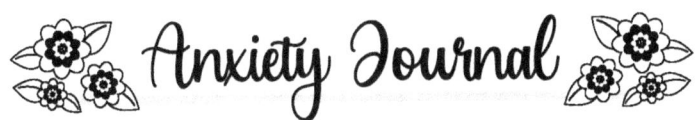

Anxiety Journal

DATE   **TIME**

PLACE   **SOURCE OF ANXIETY**

PHYSICAL SENSATIONS

NEGATIVE BELIEVES

ABOUT SITUATION ....
....

ABOUT YOUSELF ....
....

WHAT FACTS DO YOU KNOW ARE TRUE?

ABOUT SITUATION ....
....

ABOUT YOUSELF ....
....

WHAT HAPPENED?

....
....

HOW DID IT MAKE YOU FEEL?

....
....

HOW DID YOU REACT?

....
....

WHAT HELPS YOU SOOTHE YOUR ANXIETY?

....
....

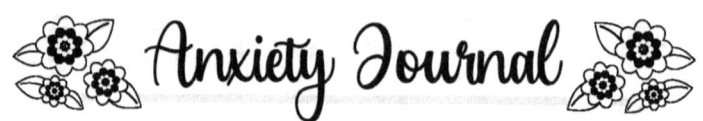

Anxiety Journal

DATE .... TIME ....

PLACE .... SOURCE OF ANXIETY ....

PHYSICAL SENSATIONS ....

NEGATIVE BELIEVES

ABOUT SITUATION ....
....

ABOUT YOUSELF ....
....

WHAT FACTS DO YOU KNOW ARE TRUE?

ABOUT SITUATION ....
....

ABOUT YOUSELF ....
....

WHAT HAPPENED?

....
....

HOW DID IT MAKE YOU FEEL?

....
....

HOW DID YOU REACT?

....
....

WHAT HELPS YOU SOOTHE YOUR ANXIETY?

....
....

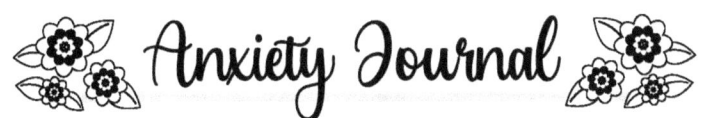

Anxiety Journal

DATE   **TIME**

PLACE   **SOURCE OF ANXIETY**

PHYSICAL SENSATIONS

NEGATIVE BELIEVES

ABOUT SITUATION ....
....

ABOUT YOUSELF ....
....

WHAT FACTS DO YOU KNOW ARE TRUE?

ABOUT SITUATION ....
....

ABOUT YOUSELF ....
....

WHAT HAPPENED?

....
....

HOW DID IT MAKE YOU FEEL?

....
....

HOW DID YOU REACT?

....
....

WHAT HELPS YOU SOOTHE YOUR ANXIETY?

....
....

Anxiety Journal

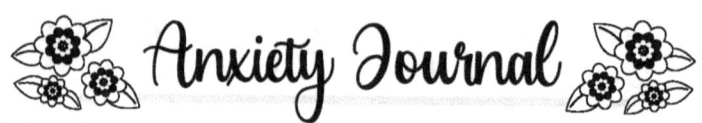

DATE TIME
PLACE SOURCE OF ANXIETY
PHYSICAL SENSATIONS

NEGATIVE BELIEVES

ABOUT SITUATION ....
....

ABOUT YOUSELF ....
....

WHAT FACTS DO YOU KNOW ARE TRUE?

ABOUT SITUATION ....
....

ABOUT YOUSELF ....
....

WHAT HAPPENED?

....
....

HOW DID IT MAKE YOU FEEL?

....
....

HOW DID YOU REACT?

....
....

WHAT HELPS YOU SOOTHE YOUR ANXIETY?

....
....

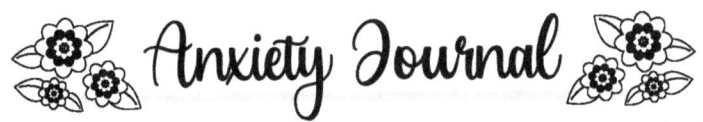

Anxiety Journal

DATE   TIME

PLACE   SOURCE OF ANXIETY

PHYSICAL SENSATIONS

NEGATIVE BELIEVES

ABOUT SITUATION ....

....

ABOUT YOUSELF ....

....

WHAT FACTS DO YOU KNOW ARE TRUE?

ABOUT SITUATION ....

....

ABOUT YOUSELF ....

....

WHAT HAPPENED?

....

....

HOW DID IT MAKE YOU FEEL?

....

....

HOW DID YOU REACT?

....

....

WHAT HELPS YOU SOOTHE YOUR ANXIETY?

....

....

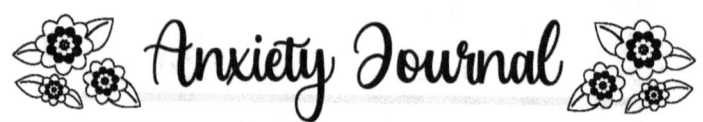

Anxiety Journal

DATE .... **TIME** ....

PLACE .... **SOURCE OF ANXIETY** ....

PHYSICAL SENSATIONS ....

NEGATIVE BELIEVES

ABOUT SITUATION ....
....

ABOUT YOUSELF ....
....

WHAT FACTS DO YOU KNOW ARE TRUE?

ABOUT SITUATION ....
....

ABOUT YOUSELF ....
....

WHAT HAPPENED?

....
....

HOW DID IT MAKE YOU FEEL?

....
....

HOW DID YOU REACT?

....
....

WHAT HELPS YOU SOOTHE YOUR ANXIETY?

....
....

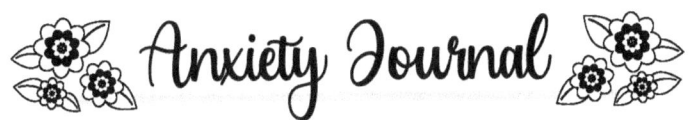

Anxiety Journal

DATE											TIME

PLACE										SOURCE OF ANXIETY

PHYSICAL SENSATIONS

NEGATIVE BELIEVES

ABOUT SITUATION ....
....

ABOUT YOUSELF ....
....

WHAT FACTS DO YOU KNOW ARE TRUE?

ABOUT SITUATION ....
....

ABOUT YOUSELF ....
....

WHAT HAPPENED?

....
....

HOW DID IT MAKE YOU FEEL?

....
....

HOW DID YOU REACT?

....
....

WHAT HELPS YOU SOOTHE YOUR ANXIETY?

....
....

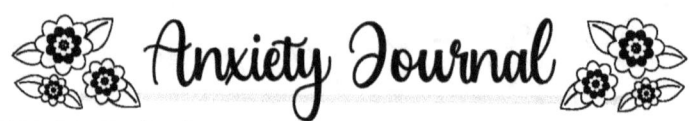

Anxiety Journal

DATE .... **TIME** ....

PLACE .... **SOURCE OF ANXIETY** ....

PHYSICAL SENSATIONS ....

NEGATIVE BELIEVES

ABOUT SITUATION ....
....

ABOUT YOUSELF ....
....

WHAT FACTS DO YOU KNOW ARE TRUE?

ABOUT SITUATION ....
....

ABOUT YOUSELF ....
....

WHAT HAPPENED?

....
....

HOW DID IT MAKE YOU FEEL?

....
....

HOW DID YOU REACT?

....
....

WHAT HELPS YOU SOOTHE YOUR ANXIETY?

....
....

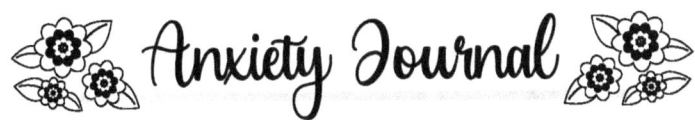

Anxiety Journal

DATE   TIME

PLACE   SOURCE OF ANXIETY

PHYSICAL SENSATIONS

NEGATIVE BELIEVES

ABOUT SITUATION ....
....
ABOUT YOUSELF ....
....

WHAT FACTS DO YOU KNOW ARE TRUE?

ABOUT SITUATION ....
....
ABOUT YOUSELF ....
....

WHAT HAPPENED?

....
....

HOW DID IT MAKE YOU FEEL?

....
....

HOW DID YOU REACT?

....
....

WHAT HELPS YOU SOOTHE YOUR ANXIETY?

....
....

Hey there!!!

We hope you enjoyed our book. As a small family company, your feedback is very important to us. Please let us know how you like our book at:

believepublisher@gmail.com

Without your voice we don't exist!

Please, support us and leave a review!

Thank you!!!

www.ingramcontent.com/pod-product-compliance
Lightning Source LLC
LaVergne TN
LVHW012001070526
838202LV00054B/4994